AFIB DIET COOKBOOK

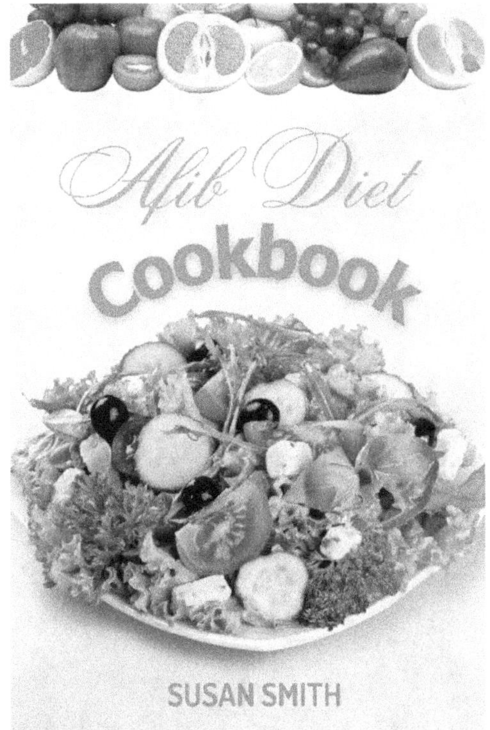

SUSAN SMITH

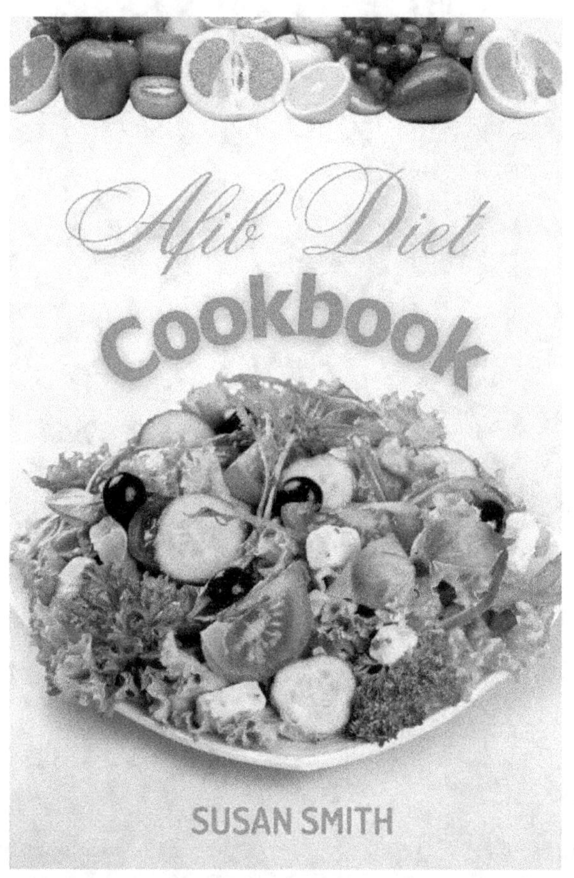
Afib Diet
Cookbook
SUSAN SMITH

TABLE OF CONTENTS

INTRODUCTION 7

CHAPTER ONE 13

Causes of AFIB disease 13

Types of AFIB disease........................15

Signs and Symptoms of AFIB Disease............16

CHAPTER TWO 19

Benefits of AFIB Disease Diet 19

AFIB Disease Preventive Measures 21

AFIB Diet Foods to Eat and Avoid 23

CHAPTER THREE 25

Healthy AFIB Diet Recipes 25

BREAKFAST RECIPES 25

1. Fruit and Yogurt Parfait.......................25

2. Oatmeal with Almonds and Berries............25

3. Avocado Toast with Poached Egg.............26

4. Chia Seed Pudding.................................27

5. Greek Yogurt and Berry Smoothie............27

7. Quinoa Breakfast Bowl..........................29

8. Cherry Almond Smoothie Bowl.................29

10. Spinach and Feta Egg Muffins 31

LUNCH RECIPES.......................................31

1. Grilled Chicken and Quinoa Salad............31

2. Salmon and Avocado Wrap......................32

3. Mediterranean Chickpea Salad.................33

4. Turkey and Veggie Lettuce Wraps.............34

5. Vegetable and Lentil Soup.......................34

6. Grilled Veggie and Goat Cheese Wrap 35

7. Tuna and White Bean Salad 36

8. Quinoa Stuffed Bell Peppers 36

9. Chicken and Vegetable Stir-Fry 37

10. Quinoa and Spinach Stuffed Portobello Mushrooms...38

DINNER RECIPES 39

1. Baked Salmon with Asparagus...................39

2. Stuffed Bell Peppers with Quinoa and Turkey 40

3. Grilled Lemon Herb Chicken 41

4. Shrimp and Zucchini Noodles 42

5. Baked Cod with Lemon and Dill 43

6. Vegetarian Stir-Fry with Tofu 43

7. Mediterranean Chickpea Stew...................44

8. Baked Chicken and Sweet Potatoes.............45

9. Eggplant and Lentil Curry 46

10. Greek Chicken and Cucumber Salad.........47

SNACK RECIPES 48

1. Apple Slices with Almond Butter...............48

2. Yogurt Parfait with Berries...........................48

3. Cucumber and Hummus Bites 49

4. Banana-Oat Energy Bites............................49

5. Avocado Toast with Cherry Tomatoes........50

6. Mixed Nuts and Dried Fruits 50

7. Carrot Sticks with Guacamole 51

8. Greek Yogurt with Honey and Walnuts 51

9. Rice Cakes with Cottage Cheese and Berries
....52

10. Frozen Grapes 52

CONCLUSION..53

INTRODUCTION

In the bustling city of Metropolis, lived a woman named Emily. She was passionate about her career, and her fast-paced lifestyle often left her little time for self-care. Over the years, Emily developed a heart condition known as atrial fibrillation (AFib). It caused irregular heartbeats, leaving her feeling anxious and fatigued.

Emily discovered the joy of cooking wholesome meals using fresh, whole ingredients. She experimented with flavorful herbs and spices that not only enhanced the taste of her dishes but also offered anti-inflammatory benefits. Turmeric became her favorite, adding a vibrant color to her meals and soothing her heart.

As she progressed on her health journey, Emily noticed positive changes. Her heartbeats became more regular, and the episodes of AFib lessened in frequency. With each passing day, she felt more invigorated and in control of her health.

Not only did Emily's diet impact her physical health, but it also had a profound effect on her emotional well-being.

The act of cooking and nourishing her body became a therapeutic practice, relieving her stress and anxiety.

Encouraged by her progress, Emily began sharing her journey with her friends and family.

She hosted heart-healthy dinner parties, introducing them to delicious recipes she had discovered. Her loved ones were amazed by her transformation and inspired to make positive changes in their own lives.

Word of Emily's success reached the local community, and she started hosting heart-healthy cooking workshops. Her passion for helping others and sharing the transformative power of a balanced diet caught the attention of the media, and soon her story was featured in newspapers and television programs.

Emily's journey not only changed her life but also touched the lives of many others. Through her dedication to a heart-healthy diet, she became an advocate for holistic health, spreading awareness about the impact of nutrition on heart conditions like AFib.

As time passed, Emily's AFib gradually faded into the background, and she embraced a vibrant and fulfilling life. She realized that a simple change in her diet had set her on a path of healing and empowerment.

Emily's story stands as a testament to the profound impact of the right diet on health and well-being. It reminds us that small, mindful choices in our daily meals can lead to significant transformations, allowing us to embrace life with a healthier heart and a renewed spirit.

Atrial Fibrillation, commonly referred to as AFib, is a prevalent and potentially serious heart condition that affects millions of people worldwide.

It is characterized by irregular and rapid heartbeats, where the heart's upper chambers (atria) quiver instead of contracting efficiently. As a result, the heart's electrical signals become chaotic, leading to an irregular heart rhythm.

In a healthy heart, a well-coordinated electrical system regulates the heartbeat, allowing it to pump blood efficiently throughout the body. However, in AFib, this electrical system becomes disrupted, causing the atria to beat rapidly and out of sync with the heart's lower chambers (ventricles).

As a consequence, the heart's pumping ability is compromised, leading to a decrease in blood flow and affecting the delivery of oxygen and nutrients to various organs and tissues.

The symptoms of AFib can vary from person to person, with some individuals experiencing noticeable signs, while others may remain asymptomatic. Common symptoms of AFib include palpitations, where the heart feels like it's fluttering, racing, or pounding.

Some individuals may also experience shortness of breath, chest discomfort, fatigue, dizziness, and lightheadedness. In more severe cases, AFib can lead to fainting or syncope.

AFib can manifest in different forms, including:

Paroxysmal AFib: This type of AFib occurs intermittently and may start and stop on its own without intervention.

Persistent AFib: In this form, the irregular heart rhythm lasts for more extended periods, usually over a week, and requires medical intervention to restore normal rhythm.

Long-standing Persistent AFib: This type of AFib occurs when the irregular rhythm lasts for more than a year.

Permanent AFib: In this form, the irregular rhythm becomes a permanent condition, and attempts to restore normal rhythm may not be successful.

While AFib itself is not life-threatening, it can lead to severe complications if left untreated. The irregular heart rhythm can cause blood to pool in the atria, increasing the risk of blood clots formation.

If a blood clot travels from the heart to the brain, it can cause a stroke, which is one of the most significant and potentially life-threatening complications of AFib. AFib can also weaken the heart muscles over time, leading to heart failure, where the heart cannot pump blood effectively to meet the body's demands.

Various factors can contribute to the development of AFib, and the exact cause may differ from person to person. Common risk factors include age (especially over 60), high blood pressure, heart disease, diabetes, obesity, sleep apnea, and a history of heart surgery or heart-related conditions.

Diagnosing AFib often involves a combination of medical history assessment, physical examination, and diagnostic tests, such as electrocardiogram (ECG or EKG), Holter monitor, event recorder, and echocardiogram.

In addition to medical treatment, lifestyle modifications play a vital role in managing AFib. Adopting a heart-healthy lifestyle, including regular exercise, a balanced diet, maintaining a healthy weight, managing stress, avoiding tobacco and excessive alcohol consumption, and adhering to medication regimens, can significantly improve the quality of life for individuals living with AFib.

Regular medical check-ups and close communication with healthcare providers are essential for individuals with AFib to monitor their condition, manage symptoms, and reduce the risk of complications.

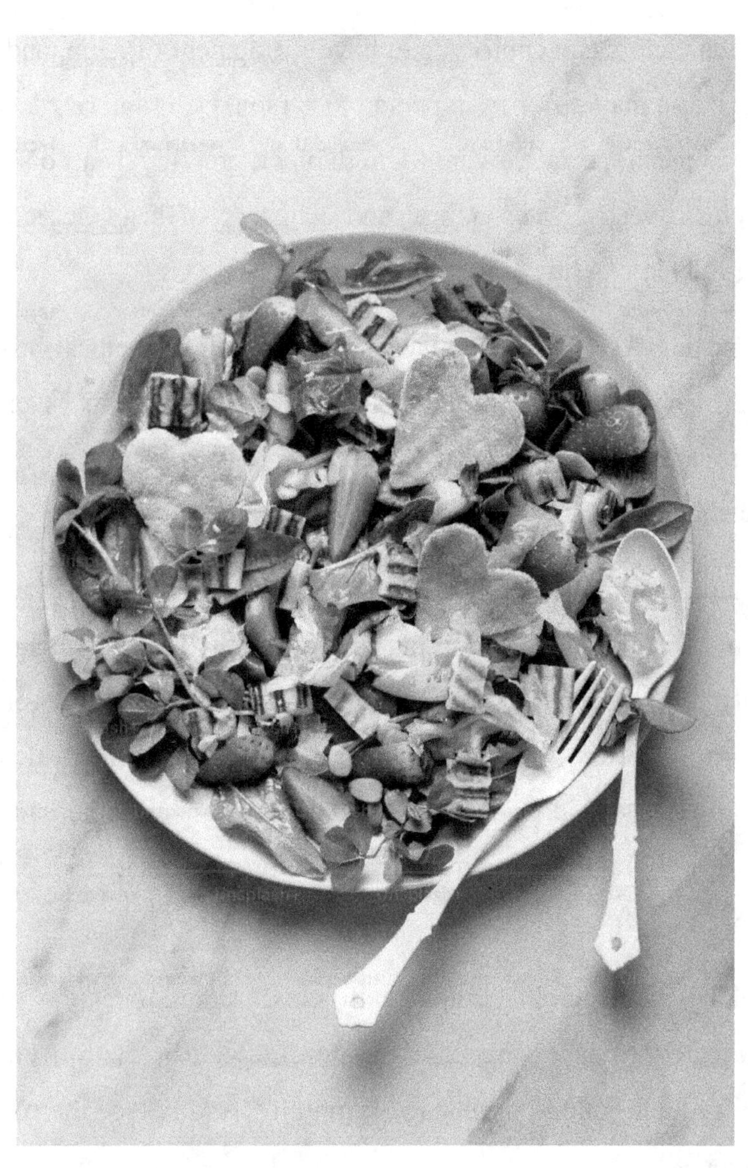

CHAPTER ONE

Causes of AFIB disease

Atrial Fibrillation (AFib) can be caused by various factors, and in many cases, the exact cause remains unclear. The development of

AFib is often multifactorial, involving a combination of underlying health conditions, lifestyle choices, and genetic predisposition. Some of the common causes and risk factors associated with AFib include:

Age: AFib becomes more common with age, especially in individuals over the age of 60. As people age, the risk of developing AFib increases due to changes in the heart's electrical system and other age-related factors.

High Blood Pressure (Hypertension): Uncontrolled high blood pressure can lead to structural changes in the heart, increasing the risk of AFib. Hypertension causes the heart to work harder to pump blood, which can strain the heart's electrical system.

Heart Diseases: Various heart conditions can contribute to AFib, such as coronary artery disease, heart valve disorders, heart failure, congenital heart defects, and prior heart surgeries. These conditions can cause structural abnormalities in the heart, disrupting its normal electrical signals.

Thyroid Disorders: Overactive or underactive thyroid glands can influence heart rhythm and increase the risk of AFib.

Chronic Conditions: Chronic conditions like diabetes, chronic kidney disease, and chronic lung diseases have been associated with an increased risk of AFib.

Obesity: Excess body weight can lead to inflammation and changes in heart structure and function, contributing to AFib.

Sleep Apnea: Sleep apnea, a condition where breathing is interrupted during sleep, has been linked to AFib due to intermittent drops in oxygen levels and stress on the heart.

Alcohol and Substance Abuse: Excessive alcohol consumption and drug abuse, particularly stimulants, can trigger AFib episodes.

Family History: Having a family history of AFib or other heart rhythm disorders may increase the risk of developing the condition.

Hyperthyroidism: An overactive thyroid gland can disrupt heart function and increase the risk of AFib.

Infections: Certain infections, such as viral infections affecting the heart (myocarditis), can contribute to the development of AFib.

Medications and Stimulants: Some medications, especially those that affect heart rhythm, can trigger AFib in susceptible individuals.

Stimulants like caffeine and certain cold medications can also provoke AFib episodes.

Types of AFIB disease

Paroxysmal AFib: Paroxysmal AFib is characterized by intermittent episodes of irregular heart rhythm that start suddenly and stop on their own within 7 days. These episodes can last for seconds, minutes, hours, or even days before returning to a normal heart rhythm.

Persistent AFib: In this type, the irregular heart rhythm lasts for more than 7 days and requires medical intervention or electrical cardioversion to restore normal heart rhythm.

Long-Standing Persistent AFib: Long-standing persistent AFib occurs when the irregular rhythm persists for over 12 months. Attempts to restore a normal heart rhythm with medications or cardioversion may not be successful.

Permanent AFib: In permanent AFib, the irregular heart rhythm becomes a constant condition, and attempts to restore a normal rhythm are not pursued or are unsuccessful. In such cases, the focus is on managing the heart rate and preventing complications.

Nonvalvular AFib: Nonvalvular AFib refers to AFib that occurs in the absence of significant heart valve abnormalities. It is the most common type of AFib.

Valvular AFib: Valvular AFib is associated with heart valve disorders, such as mitral valve stenosis or mechanical heart valve replacements. It requires careful management and may have different treatment considerations.

Lone AFib: Lone AFib occurs in individuals under the age of 60 who have no other significant heart conditions or risk factors. It is less common and may have a lower risk of complications compared to AFib in older individuals with multiple risk factors.

Signs and Symptoms of AFIB Disease

Atrial Fibrillation (AFib) can present with a range of signs and symptoms, which can vary from person to person. Some individuals with AFib may experience noticeable symptoms, while others may not have any noticeable signs. Common signs and symptoms of AFib include:

Palpitations: Palpitations are the most common symptom of AFib. Individuals may feel that their heart is fluttering, racing, or pounding irregularly.

Irregular Heartbeat: AFib causes the heart's rhythm to be irregular. Instead of the usual steady and coordinated heartbeat, the heart's contractions become chaotic and irregular.

Fatigue: AFib can lead to decreased blood flow to the body, resulting in fatigue and reduced energy levels.

Shortness of Breath: Some individuals with AFib may experience shortness of breath, especially during physical activity or exertion.

Dizziness or Lightheadedness: Insufficient blood flow to the brain due to AFib can cause dizziness or lightheadedness.

Chest Discomfort: AFib may be associated with mild chest discomfort or a sensation of pressure in the chest.

Weakness: Muscle weakness or feeling weak can be a symptom of AFib, especially when combined with other signs.

Confusion or Brain Fog: In some cases, AFib can affect blood flow to the brain, leading to confusion or difficulty concentrating.

Fainting or Syncope: In more severe cases, AFib can cause a sudden drop in blood pressure, leading to fainting or syncope.

It is essential to recognize these signs and symptoms and seek medical attention promptly if they occur, especially if they are persistent or severe.

Some individuals may experience "silent AFib," where they have the irregular heart rhythm without noticeable symptoms.

In such cases, AFib may be detected during routine medical check-ups or through an electrocardiogram (ECG) test.

It is important to diagnose and manage AFib early to prevent potential complications, such as blood clots, stroke, and heart failure.

Healthcare providers may use various diagnostic tests, such as ECG, Holter monitor, event recorder, or echocardiogram, to confirm the presence of AFib and determine its type and severity.

If you or someone you know experiences any signs or symptoms of AFib, it is crucial to seek medical evaluation to assess heart health and discuss appropriate management options.

Early detection and timely treatment can lead to better outcomes and improved quality of life for individuals living with AFib.

CHAPTER TWO

Benefits of AFIB Disease Diet

It's important to clarify that there is no specific "AFib disease diet" as such. However, adopting a heart-healthy diet can provide several benefits for individuals with Atrial Fibrillation (AFib) and those at risk of heart-related conditions. A heart-healthy diet may include the following benefits:

Cardiovascular Support: A heart-healthy diet focuses on whole foods that are rich in nutrients, such as fruits, vegetables, whole grains, lean proteins, and healthy fats. These foods provide essential vitamins and minerals that support cardiovascular health and overall well-being.

Blood Pressure Management: Many heart-healthy foods, such as fruits and vegetables, are low in sodium, which can help manage blood pressure levels. High blood pressure is a risk factor for AFib, so maintaining healthy blood pressure is essential for heart health.

Weight Management: A heart-healthy diet emphasizes portion control and the consumption of nutrient-dense foods, which can aid in weight management. Maintaining a healthy weight reduces the strain on the heart and may help manage AFib symptoms.

Blood Sugar Control: For individuals with diabetes or prediabetes, managing blood sugar levels is vital. A heart-healthy diet that includes whole grains, non-starchy vegetables, and healthy fats can support blood sugar control.

Cholesterol Reduction: Foods rich in soluble fiber, such as oats, beans, and fruits, can help lower LDL cholesterol levels, reducing the risk of heart disease and related complications.

Inflammation Reduction: Certain heart-healthy foods, such as fatty fish rich in omega-3 fatty acids and colorful fruits and vegetables, contain anti-inflammatory properties that may help reduce inflammation in the body.

Antioxidant Benefits: Many heart-healthy foods are rich in antioxidants, which help neutralize harmful free radicals in the body and may protect the heart and blood vessels from damage.

Fluid Balance: For individuals with AFib, maintaining a proper fluid balance is essential.

A heart-healthy diet that includes foods with moderate sodium content can help manage fluid retention.

Improved Digestion: A heart-healthy diet that includes fiber-rich foods can promote healthy digestion and regular bowel movements.

Overall Well-Being: A balanced and nutritious diet can contribute to better energy levels, improved mood, and overall well-being.

AFIB Disease Preventive Measures

Maintain a Healthy Lifestyle: Adopting a healthy lifestyle can significantly reduce the risk of AFib. This includes eating a balanced and heart-healthy diet, engaging in regular physical activity, managing stress, getting enough sleep, and avoiding tobacco and excessive alcohol consumption.

Manage High Blood Pressure: High blood pressure is a significant risk factor for AFib. Regularly monitor blood pressure and work with healthcare providers to manage it through lifestyle changes, medications, or a combination of both.

Control Blood Sugar: For individuals with diabetes or prediabetes, managing blood sugar levels is crucial. Consistent blood sugar control can reduce the risk of developing AFib and prevent complications.

Maintain a Healthy Weight: Being overweight or obese can increase the risk of AFib. Achieving and maintaining a healthy weight through a combination of a balanced diet and regular exercise can reduce this risk.

Stay Active: Engaging in regular physical activity can support heart health and reduce the risk of AFib.

Aim for at least 150 minutes of moderate-intensity aerobic exercise or 75 minutes of vigorous-intensity exercise per week, along with muscle-strengthening activities on two or more days per week.

Limit Caffeine and Stimulant Intake: Excessive caffeine and stimulant consumption can trigger AFib episodes in some individuals. Limiting or avoiding these substances may be beneficial.

Manage Stress: Chronic stress can contribute to the development of AFib.

Practice stress-reduction techniques such as meditation, deep breathing exercises, yoga, or engaging in hobbies to promote relaxation.

Get Regular Check-ups: Regular medical check-ups are essential for detecting and managing AFib or other heart-related conditions.

Routine visits with healthcare providers can help monitor heart health and identify any potential issues early on.

Follow Medical Advice: If diagnosed with AFib or any heart-related condition, it is crucial to follow the prescribed medical treatment and management plan. Take medications as directed, attend regular follow-ups, and communicate openly with healthcare providers.

Limit Alcohol Intake: Excessive alcohol consumption can trigger AFib episodes and increase the risk of complications. If you drink alcohol, do so in moderation as per the recommendations of healthcare providers.

Treat Underlying Conditions: Managing and treating underlying health conditions, such as sleep apnea, thyroid disorders, and chronic lung diseases, can help reduce the risk of AFib.

AFIB Diet Foods to Eat and Avoid

When managing Atrial Fibrillation (AFib), it's essential to focus on a heart-healthy diet that supports overall cardiovascular health. Here are some recommended foods to eat and foods to avoid for individuals with AFib:

Foods to Eat:

Fruits and Vegetables: Include a variety of colorful fruits and vegetables in your diet. They are rich in vitamins, minerals, fiber, and antioxidants that support heart health.

Whole Grains: Opt for whole grains such as oats, quinoa, brown rice, and whole wheat bread. These provide complex carbohydrates, fiber, and essential nutrients.

Lean Proteins: Choose lean sources of protein like skinless poultry, fish (especially fatty fish high in omega-3 fatty acids), legumes, tofu, and nuts. These options are lower in saturated fat and support heart health.

Healthy Fats: Incorporate sources of healthy fats like avocados, nuts, seeds, and olive oil. These fats are beneficial for heart health and can help reduce inflammation.

Low-Fat Dairy: If you consume dairy, choose low-fat or non-fat options like skim milk, low-fat yogurt, and reduced-fat cheese.

Beans and Lentils: These are excellent sources of protein, fiber, and various nutrients and are heart-healthy choices.

Water: Staying hydrated with water is essential for overall health, including heart health.

Foods to Limit or Avoid:

Sodium: Reduce your intake of salt and foods high in sodium, as excessive sodium can contribute to high blood pressure. Avoid processed foods, canned soups, and salty snacks.

Saturated and Trans Fats: Limit foods high in saturated fats such as fatty cuts of meat, full-fat dairy products, and fried foods. Avoid trans fats found in many processed and fried foods.

Sugary Foods and Beverages: Minimize consumption of sugary foods and drinks, including sodas, juices, and desserts.

CHAPTER THREE

Healthy AFIB Diet Recipes

BREAKFAST RECIPES

1. Fruit and Yogurt Parfait

Ingredients:

- 1 cup low-fat yogurt
- 1/2 cup mixed berries (strawberries, blueberries, raspberries)
- 2 tablespoons granola
- 1 teaspoon honey (optional)

Instructions:

- In a glass or bowl, layer the yogurt, mixed berries, and granola.
- Drizzle with honey if desired.

Cooking Time: 5 minutes

2. Oatmeal with Almonds and Berries

Ingredients:

- 1/2 cup rolled oats
- 1 cup almond milk
- 1 tablespoon chopped almonds

- 1/2 cup mixed berries

- 1 teaspoon honey (optional)

Instructions:

- In a saucepan, combine oats and almond milk. Cook over medium heat until the oats are tender.

- Top with chopped almonds, mixed berries, and drizzle with honey if desired.

Cooking Time: 10 minutes

3. Avocado Toast with Poached Egg

Ingredients:

- 1 slice whole-grain bread

- 1/2 ripe avocado, mashed

- 1 poached egg

- Salt and pepper to taste

Instructions:

- Toast the bread until lightly browned.

- Spread mashed avocado on the toast and top with the poached egg.

- Season with salt and pepper to taste.

Cooking Time: 15 minutes

4. Chia Seed Pudding

Ingredients:

- 2 tablespoons chia seeds
- 1 cup almond milk
- 1/2 teaspoon vanilla extract
- 1/2 cup sliced bananas
- 1 tablespoon chopped walnuts

Instructions:

- In a bowl, mix chia seeds, almond milk, and vanilla extract. Stir well and refrigerate overnight.
- In the morning, top with sliced bananas and chopped walnuts.

Cooking Time: Overnight + 5 minutes

5. Greek Yogurt and Berry Smoothie

Ingredients:

- 1 cup Greek yogurt
- 1/2 cup mixed berries
- 1 tablespoon honey
- 1/2 cup almond milk

Instructions:

- In a blender, combine Greek yogurt, mixed berries, honey, and almond milk.
- Blend until smooth and creamy.
- Cooking Time: 5 minutes
- 6. Egg White Veggie Omelette

Ingredients:

- 3 egg whites
- 1/4 cup diced bell peppers
- 1/4 cup diced tomatoes
- 1/4 cup chopped spinach
- 1 tablespoon chopped fresh herbs (parsley, basil, or chives)

Instructions:

- In a bowl, whisk the egg whites until frothy.
- In a non-stick skillet, sauté the bell peppers, tomatoes, and spinach for a few minutes.
- Pour the egg whites over the veggies and cook until set. Sprinkle with fresh herbs.

Cooking Time: 10 minutes

7. Quinoa Breakfast Bowl

Ingredients:

- 1/2 cup cooked quinoa
- 1/4 cup sliced almonds
- 1/2 cup sliced peaches or berries
- 1 tablespoon honey (optional)

Instructions:

- In a bowl, combine cooked quinoa, sliced almonds, and sliced peaches or berries.
- Drizzle with honey if desired.
- Cooking Time: 15 minutes (if quinoa is not pre-cooked)

8. Cherry Almond Smoothie Bowl

Ingredients:

- 1 cup frozen cherries
- 1/2 cup almond milk
- 1 tablespoon almond butter
- 1 tablespoon chia seeds
- Toppings: sliced bananas, chopped almonds

Instructions:

- In a blender, blend frozen cherries, almond milk, almond butter, and chia seeds until smooth.

- Pour the smoothie into a bowl and top with sliced bananas and chopped almonds.

- Cooking Time: 5 minutes

- 9. Whole Grain Pancakes with Berries

- Ingredients:

- 1/2 cup whole wheat flour

- 1/2 cup almond milk

- 1 tablespoon honey

- 1 teaspoon baking powder

- 1/4 cup mixed berries

Instructions:

- In a bowl, mix whole wheat flour, almond milk, honey, and baking powder until well combined.

- Heat a non-stick skillet over medium heat. Pour 1/4 cup of the batter onto the skillet to form a pancake.

- Cook until bubbles form on the surface, then flip and cook until golden brown.

- Serve with mixed berries on top.

Cooking Time: 15 minutes

10. Spinach and Feta Egg Muffins

Ingredients:

- 4 eggs

- 1/2 cup chopped spinach

- 1/4 cup crumbled feta cheese

- Salt and pepper to taste

Instructions:

- Preheat the oven to 350°F (175°C) and grease a muffin tin.

- In a bowl, whisk the eggs and season with salt and pepper.

- Stir in chopped spinach and feta cheese.

- Pour the mixture into the muffin tin, filling each cup about two-thirds full.

- Bake for 15-20 minutes or until the egg muffins are set and golden brown.

Cooking Time: 20 minutes

LUNCH RECIPES

1. Grilled Chicken and Quinoa Salad

Ingredients:

- 1 cup cooked quinoa

- 4 ounces grilled chicken breast, sliced

- 1 cup mixed salad greens

- 1/4 cup cherry tomatoes, halved

- 1/4 cup cucumber, diced

- 2 tablespoons balsamic vinaigrette dressing

Instructions:

- In a bowl, combine cooked quinoa, grilled chicken, mixed salad greens, cherry tomatoes, and cucumber.

- Drizzle with balsamic vinaigrette dressing and toss to combine.

Cooking Time: 15 minutes (if quinoa is not pre-cooked)

2. Salmon and Avocado Wrap

Ingredients:

- 4 ounces grilled or baked salmon

- 1 whole-grain tortilla or wrap

- 1/4 ripe avocado, sliced

- 1 cup baby spinach leaves

- 1 tablespoon Greek yogurt dill sauce (Greek yogurt mixed with dill and lemon juice)

Instructions:

- Lay the whole-grain tortilla flat and spread the Greek yogurt dill sauce over it.

- Place grilled salmon, sliced avocado, and baby spinach leaves on the tortilla.

- Roll the tortilla into a wrap and secure with toothpicks if needed.

Cooking Time: 15 minutes (if salmon is not pre-cooked)

3. Mediterranean Chickpea Salad

Ingredients:

- 1 can (15 ounces) chickpeas, drained and rinsed

- 1/2 cup cherry tomatoes, halved

- 1/4 cup diced cucumber

- 1/4 cup diced red onion

- 2 tablespoons crumbled feta cheese

- 1 tablespoon olive oil

- 1 tablespoon lemon juice

- 1 teaspoon dried oregano

Instructions:

- In a bowl, combine chickpeas, cherry tomatoes, cucumber, red onion, and feta cheese.

- Drizzle with olive oil and lemon juice. Sprinkle dried oregano on top and toss to mix.

Cooking Time: 10 minutes

4. Turkey and Veggie Lettuce Wraps

Ingredients:

- 4 large lettuce leaves (such as romaine or iceberg)
- 4 ounces deli turkey slices
- 1/4 cup shredded carrots
- 1/4 cup sliced bell peppers
- 2 tablespoons hummus

Instructions:

- Lay the lettuce leaves flat and top each with deli turkey slices, shredded carrots, and sliced bell peppers.
- Spread hummus on top of the veggies.
- Roll the lettuce leaves into wraps and secure with toothpicks if needed.

Cooking Time: 10 minutes

5. Vegetable and Lentil Soup

Ingredients:

- 1 cup cooked lentils
- 1 cup mixed vegetables (carrots, celery, zucchini, etc.)
- 4 cups low-sodium vegetable broth
- 1 teaspoon olive oil
- 1/2 teaspoon dried thyme

- Salt and pepper to taste

Instructions:

- In a pot, heat olive oil and sauté mixed vegetables until tender.
- Add cooked lentils, vegetable broth, dried thyme, salt, and pepper.
- Simmer for 15-20 minutes or until the flavors meld together.

Cooking Time: 25 minutes (if lentils are not pre-cooked)

6. Grilled Veggie and Goat Cheese Wrap

Ingredients:

- 1 whole-grain tortilla or wrap
- 1/2 cup grilled vegetables (bell peppers, eggplant, zucchini, etc.)
- 2 tablespoons crumbled goat cheese
- 1/4 cup baby spinach leaves
- 1 tablespoon balsamic glaze

Instructions:

- Lay the whole-grain tortilla flat and sprinkle crumbled goat cheese on it.
- Add grilled vegetables and baby spinach leaves on top.
- Drizzle with balsamic glaze and roll the tortilla into a wrap.

Cooking Time: 15 minutes (if vegetables are not pre-cooked)

7. Tuna and White Bean Salad

Ingredients:

- 1 can (5 ounces) tuna, drained
- 1 can (15 ounces) white beans, drained and rinsed
- 1/4 cup chopped red onion
- 1/4 cup chopped bell peppers
- 2 tablespoons chopped fresh parsley
- 1 tablespoon olive oil
- 1 tablespoon lemon juice
- Salt and pepper to taste

Instructions:

- In a bowl, combine tuna, white beans, red onion, bell peppers, and fresh parsley.
- Drizzle with olive oil and lemon juice. Season with salt and pepper and toss to mix.

Cooking Time: 10 minutes

8. Quinoa Stuffed Bell Peppers

Ingredients:

- 2 large bell peppers (any color)
- 1 cup cooked quinoa

- 1/2 cup black beans, drained and rinsed

- 1/4 cup diced tomatoes

- 1/4 cup diced red onion

- 1/4 cup shredded cheddar cheese (optional)

Instructions:

- Preheat the oven to 375°F (190°C). Cut the tops off the bell peppers and remove the seeds.

- In a bowl, mix cooked quinoa, black beans, diced tomatoes, red onion, and shredded cheddar cheese (if using).

- Stuff the bell peppers with the quinoa mixture and place them in a baking dish.

- Bake for 20-25 minutes or until the bell peppers are tender.

Cooking Time: 30 minutes (if quinoa is not pre-cooked)

9. Chicken and Vegetable Stir-Fry

Ingredients:

- 4 ounces cooked chicken breast, sliced

- 1 cup mixed stir-fry vegetables (broccoli, bell peppers, snow peas, etc.)

- 1 tablespoon low-sodium soy sauce

- 1 teaspoon sesame oil

- 1/2 teaspoon minced garlic

- 1/4 teaspoon grated ginger

Instructions:

- In a skillet or wok, heat sesame oil over medium-high heat.
- Add garlic and ginger, followed by mixed stir-fry vegetables. Cook for a few minutes until vegetables are tender-crisp.
- Add sliced chicken and low-sodium soy sauce. Stir-fry for another minute or until chicken is heated through.

Cooking Time: 15 minutes (if chicken is not pre-cooked)

10. Quinoa and Spinach Stuffed Portobello Mushrooms

Ingredients:

- 2 large Portobello mushrooms
- 1 cup cooked quinoa
- 1 cup fresh spinach leaves
- 1/4 cup diced tomatoes
- 1/4 cup crumbled feta cheese
- 1 tablespoon balsamic glaze

Instructions:

- Preheat the oven to 375°F (190°C). Clean the Portobello mushrooms and remove the stems.

- In a bowl, mix cooked quinoa, fresh spinach leaves, diced tomatoes, and crumbled feta cheese.

- Stuff the Portobello mushrooms with the quinoa mixture and place them on a baking sheet.

- Bake for 20-25 minutes or until the mushrooms are tender and the filling is heated through.

- Drizzle with balsamic glaze before serving.

Cooking Time: 30 minutes (if quinoa is not pre-cooked)

DINNER RECIPES

1. Baked Salmon with Asparagus

Ingredients:

- 4 ounces salmon fillet

- 1/2 bunch asparagus spears

- 1 tablespoon olive oil

- 1 lemon, sliced

- Salt and pepper to taste

Instructions:

- Preheat the oven to 375°F (190°C). Place the salmon fillet on a baking sheet.

- Arrange asparagus spears around the salmon.

- Drizzle olive oil over the salmon and asparagus. Season with salt and pepper.

- Place lemon slices on top of the salmon.

- Bake for 15-20 minutes or until the salmon is cooked through and the asparagus is tender.

Cooking Time: 20 minutes

2. Stuffed Bell Peppers with Quinoa and Turkey

Ingredients:

- 2 large bell peppers (any color)

- 1 cup cooked quinoa

- 4 ounces ground turkey, cooked and seasoned

- 1/4 cup diced tomatoes

- 1/4 cup diced zucchini

- 1/4 cup shredded mozzarella cheese (optional)

Instructions:

- Preheat the oven to 375°F (190°C). Cut the tops off the bell peppers and remove the seeds.

- In a bowl, mix cooked quinoa, seasoned ground turkey, diced tomatoes, and diced zucchini.

- Stuff the bell peppers with the quinoa and turkey mixture.

- Sprinkle shredded mozzarella cheese on top if using.

- Bake for 25-30 minutes or until the bell peppers are tender and the filling is heated through.

Cooking Time: 35 minutes (if quinoa and turkey are not pre-cooked)

3. Grilled Lemon Herb Chicken

Ingredients:

- 4 ounces chicken breast

- Juice of 1 lemon

- 1 tablespoon olive oil

- 1 teaspoon dried herbs (such as oregano, thyme, or rosemary)

- Salt and pepper to taste

Instructions:

- In a bowl, combine lemon juice, olive oil, dried herbs, salt, and pepper.

- Add the chicken breast to the marinade and let it sit for at least 30 minutes.

- Preheat the grill to medium-high heat.

- Grill the chicken for 6-8 minutes per side or until it's cooked through and no longer pink in the center.

Cooking Time: 20 minutes (including marinating time)

4. Shrimp and Zucchini Noodles

Ingredients:

- 4 ounces shrimp, peeled and deveined
- 2 zucchini, spiralized into noodles
- 1 tablespoon olive oil
- 2 cloves garlic, minced
- 1/4 teaspoon red pepper flakes (optional)
- 1 tablespoon chopped fresh parsley

Instructions:

- In a skillet, heat olive oil over medium heat. Add minced garlic and red pepper flakes (if using).
- Add shrimp to the skillet and cook for 2-3 minutes per side or until they turn pink and opaque.
- Add zucchini noodles to the skillet and toss with the shrimp and garlic.
- Cook for 1-2 minutes or until the zucchini noodles are tender.
- Sprinkle chopped fresh parsley on top before serving.

Cooking Time: 10 minutes

5. Baked Cod with Lemon and Dill

Ingredients:

- 4 ounces cod fillet
- Juice of 1 lemon
- 1 tablespoon olive oil
- 1 teaspoon dried dill
- Salt and pepper to taste

Instructions:

- Preheat the oven to 375°F (190°C). Place the cod fillet on a baking sheet.
- In a small bowl, mix lemon juice, olive oil, dried dill, salt, and pepper.
- Drizzle the lemon-dill mixture over the cod fillet.
- Bake for 12-15 minutes or until the cod is flaky and cooked through.

Cooking Time: 15 minutes

6. Vegetarian Stir-Fry with Tofu

Ingredients:

- 4 ounces firm tofu, cubed
- 1 cup mixed stir-fry vegetables (broccoli, bell peppers, snap peas, etc.)

- 2 tablespoons low-sodium soy sauce

- 1 tablespoon hoisin sauce

- 1 teaspoon sesame oil

- 1/4 teaspoon grated ginger

Instructions:

- In a non-stick skillet or wok, heat sesame oil over medium-high heat.

- Add cubed tofu and cook until lightly browned on all sides.

- Add mixed stir-fry vegetables and grated ginger. Stir-fry for a few minutes until the vegetables are tender-crisp.

- Stir in low-sodium soy sauce and hoisin sauce. Cook for another minute.

Cooking Time: 15 minutes

7. Mediterranean Chickpea Stew

Ingredients:

- 1 can (15 ounces) chickpeas, drained and rinsed

- 1 can (14 ounces) diced tomatoes

- 1 cup vegetable broth

- 1/4 cup chopped red onion

- 1/4 cup chopped bell peppers

- 1/4 cup sliced black olives

- 1 tablespoon olive oil

- 1 teaspoon dried oregano

- Salt and pepper to taste

Instructions:

- In a pot, heat olive oil over medium heat. Add chopped red onion and bell peppers. Sauté until softened.

- Add chickpeas, diced tomatoes, vegetable broth, dried oregano, salt, and pepper.

- Simmer for 10-15 minutes or until the stew thickens slightly.

- Stir in sliced black olives before serving.

Cooking Time: 20 minutes

8. Baked Chicken and Sweet Potatoes

Ingredients:

- 4 ounces chicken breast

- 1 small sweet potato, peeled and diced

- 1 tablespoon olive oil

- 1 teaspoon dried thyme

- Salt and pepper to taste

Instructions:

- Preheat the oven to 375°F (190°C). Place the chicken breast on a baking sheet.

- Toss diced sweet potatoes with olive oil, dried thyme, salt, and pepper.

- Arrange the sweet potatoes around the chicken on the baking sheet.

- Bake for 20-25 minutes or until the chicken is cooked through and the sweet potatoes are tender.

Cooking Time: 25 minutes

9. Eggplant and Lentil Curry

Ingredients:

- 1 cup cooked lentils

- 1 small eggplant, diced

- 1 can (14 ounces) coconut milk

- 1 tablespoon curry powder

- 1/4 teaspoon turmeric

- Salt and pepper to taste

Instructions:

- In a pot, combine cooked lentils, diced eggplant, coconut milk, curry powder, turmeric, salt, and pepper.

- Bring the mixture to a simmer and cook for 15-20 minutes or until the eggplant is tender.

- Serve over brown rice or quinoa if desired.

Cooking Time: 25 minutes (if lentils are not pre-cooked)

10. Greek Chicken and Cucumber Salad

Ingredients:

- 4 ounces grilled or baked chicken breast, sliced
- 1 cup cucumber, diced
- 1/4 cup cherry tomatoes, halved
- 1/4 cup sliced red onion
- 2 tablespoons crumbled feta cheese
- 1 tablespoon olive oil
- 1 tablespoon lemon juice
- 1 teaspoon dried oregano

Instructions:

- In a bowl, combine sliced grilled chicken, diced cucumber, cherry tomatoes, sliced red onion, and crumbled feta cheese.
- Drizzle with olive oil and lemon juice. Sprinkle dried oregano on top and toss to mix.

Cooking Time: 10 minutes (if chicken is not pre-cooked)

SNACK RECIPES

1. Apple Slices with Almond Butter

Ingredients:

- 1 medium apple, sliced
- 2 tablespoons almond butter

Instructions:

- Wash and slice the apple into thin pieces.
- Serve the apple slices with almond butter for dipping.

Preparation Time: 5 minutes

2. Yogurt Parfait with Berries

Ingredients:

- 1 cup low-fat plain yogurt
- 1/2 cup mixed berries (strawberries, blueberries, raspberries)
- 2 tablespoons granola (optional)

Instructions:

- In a glass or bowl, layer the yogurt, mixed berries, and granola (if using).
- Repeat the layers until all the ingredients are used.

Preparation Time: 5 minutes

3. Cucumber and Hummus Bites

Ingredients:

- 1 medium cucumber, sliced
- 1/4 cup hummus

Instructions:

- Wash and slice the cucumber into rounds.
- Top each cucumber slice with a small dollop of hummus.

Preparation Time: 5 minutes

4. Banana-Oat Energy Bites

Ingredients:

- 1 ripe banana, mashed
- 1 cup rolled oats
- 2 tablespoons almond butter
- 1/4 teaspoon cinnamon

Instructions:

- In a bowl, mix mashed banana, rolled oats, almond butter, and cinnamon until well combined.
- Shape the mixture into small energy bites.

Preparation Time: 10 minutes

5. Avocado Toast with Cherry Tomatoes

Ingredients:

- 1 slice whole-grain bread, toasted
- 1/2 ripe avocado, mashed
- 1/4 cup cherry tomatoes, halved
- Pinch of salt and pepper

Instructions:

- Spread the mashed avocado on the toasted bread.
- Top with halved cherry tomatoes and season with salt and pepper.

Preparation Time: 5 minutes

6. Mixed Nuts and Dried Fruits

Ingredients:

- 1/4 cup mixed nuts (almonds, walnuts, cashews)
- 1/4 cup mixed dried fruits (raisins, apricots, cranberries)

Instructions:

- Combine the mixed nuts and dried fruits in a bowl.
- Mix well and enjoy!

Preparation Time: 2 minutes

7. Carrot Sticks with Guacamole

Ingredients:

- 2 medium carrots, cut into sticks
- 1/4 cup guacamole

Instructions:

- Wash and cut the carrots into sticks.
- Serve with guacamole for dipping.

Preparation Time: 5 minutes

8. Greek Yogurt with Honey and Walnuts

Ingredients:

- 1 cup low-fat Greek yogurt
- 1 tablespoon honey
- 2 tablespoons chopped walnuts

Instructions:

- In a bowl, mix the Greek yogurt with honey.
- Sprinkle chopped walnuts on top before serving.

Preparation Time: 5 minutes

9. Rice Cakes with Cottage Cheese and Berries

Ingredients:

- 2 rice cakes
- 1/2 cup low-fat cottage cheese
- 1/2 cup mixed berries (strawberries, blueberries, raspberries)

Instructions:

- Spread cottage cheese on each rice cake.
- Top with mixed berries.

Preparation Time: 5 minutes

10. Frozen Grapes

Ingredients:

- 1 cup grapes, frozen

Instructions:

- Wash and pat dry the grapes.
- Place the grapes in the freezer for at least 2 hours or until frozen.
- Enjoy the refreshing and naturally sweet frozen grapes!

Preparation Time: 2 hours (freezing time)

CONCLUSION

Adopting an AFib-friendly diet can have a profound impact on managing and improving the quality of life for individuals with Atrial Fibrillation.

By incorporating heart-healthy foods and making mindful dietary choices, you can promote heart health, reduce inflammation, and support overall well-being.

Throughout this journey, we have explored a diverse range of delicious and nutritious recipes specially crafted to accommodate AFib dietary recommendations.

From wholesome breakfast options to satisfying dinners and delightful snacks, these recipes demonstrate that maintaining a heart-healthy diet doesn't mean sacrificing flavor or enjoyment.

By prioritizing nutrient-dense foods like leafy greens, colorful vegetables, lean proteins, and heart-healthy fats, you can help manage AFib risk factors and promote a healthier heart rhythm.

Reducing sodium intake, limiting processed foods, and staying hydrated also play crucial roles in supporting your heart health.

Remember, a well-balanced diet is just one part of a holistic approach to managing AFib.

Always consult with your healthcare provider or a registered dietitian for personalized advice tailored to your unique health needs and medical history.

With determination, commitment, and the right dietary choices, you can take charge of your health and support a better future for yourself or your loved ones living with Atrial Fibrillation.

Embrace the power of food to nourish your body and empower your heart on your journey to a heart-healthy lifestyle.

Here's to a vibrant and fulfilling life, enriched by the vitality and wellness that comes with making nutritious choices and embracing a heart-healthy diet.

Let your heart be your guide, and may the nourishment you provide your body pave the way for a healthier, happier tomorrow.

www.ingramcontent.com/pod-product-compliance
Lightning Source LLC
Chambersburg PA
CBHW051707250726

48653CB00007B/2899